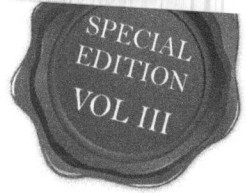
SPECIAL EDITION VOL III

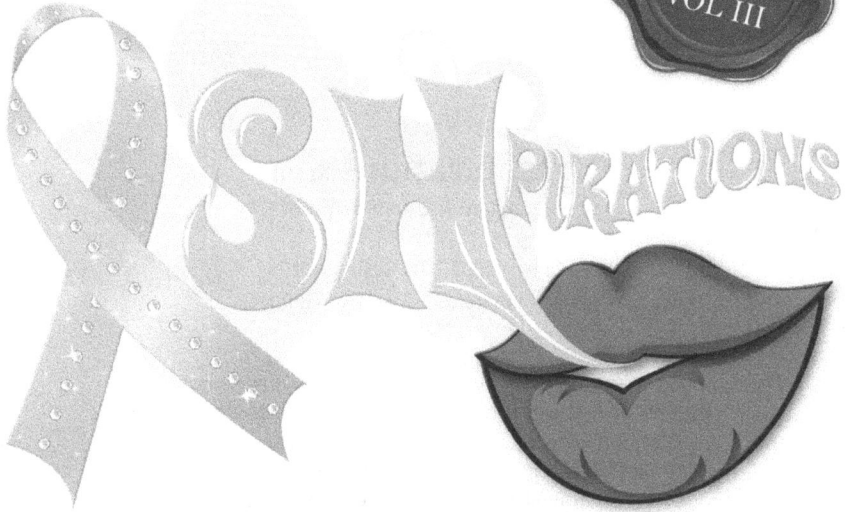

In Memoriam

Celebration of Life

'Ishpirations Vol III
In Memoriam & Celebration of Life

Copyright © 2012 Regina Griffin

Cover and interior design by Ted Ruybal

ISBN 13: 978-0-6156990-4-2

ISBN 10: 0-6156990-4-9

LCCN: 2012917080

First Edition

1 2 3 4 5 6 7 8 9 10

Inspiration/Healing

For information, please contact:

GRIFFIN SCOTT
PRESS

www.dishtheish.com

In
Celebration
of
Angela Neloms

You epitomize what it means to be a warrior.

Your walk, strength and entrepreneurial spirit are extraordinary.

You never once broke stride in your healing.

You are a fighter.

You are courageous.

You are an Ishpiration.

Cancer didn't beat you.

YOU BEAT IT!

We love you,
Regina & Mark

About the Book

Today, 111 women in the United States will die from breast cancer, according to American Cancer Society statistics. It is the second most prevalent cancer among women. Approximately 1 in 8 will be diagnosed in her lifetime, and 1 in 36 has the chance of dying from the disease. There are over 100,000 new cases diagnosed every year. In 2012, the American Cancer Society predicts the number will more than double to 226,870 cases.

"Ishpirations—In Memoriam and Celebration of Life" is VOL III of the bestselling "Ish" series. This installment is dedicated to breast cancer warriors who have lost or won the formidable battle against breast cancer. The book is filled with 140 inspirational one-liner quips that will inspire, motivate, memorialize and celebrate breast cancer's lost souls and survivors. Some of the ishpirations are accompanied by real-life, heartfelt dedications from friends and family members of beloved survivors and transitioned souls. Ishpirations will inspire readers, soothe the spirit and warm the heart.

Acknowledgements

Yes, it's true. My name is Regina Griffin, and I have a black belt in the art of 'Ish. I received my Bachelors of Science from Gmail, an MBA from Facebook and most recently, an honorary PhD from Twitter. Dishing the 'Ish is truly what I do.

This time around though, I've been led to dish for a cause—breast cancer prevention and awareness. Only second to lung cancer, breast cancer is the leading cause of death of women in the United States. Last year, the disease stole the lives of an estimated 39,510 women.

Angela Neloms, is my inspiration for this book. She was diagnosed with breast cancer in 2011, and at the time of publishing has been cancer free for over 12 months. She is the first woman I have personally known to battle breast cancer. Her fight has been quiet, powerful, relentless and graceful. Seeing her fight and maintain her everyday life made me curious and spiritually committed to the cause. I had to get involved, so I picked up the phone, called my local branch of Susan G. Komen and said "I'm in," and the idea of Ishpirations followed.

Respectively, this book is homage to all battlers of the senseless disease. You will find heartfelt memorials and celebrations scattered throughout the book. They are living tributes from friends and family members of the warriors who have lost and survived breast cancer. There are so many who must be thanked. Without their support, and dedication the task of completing this edition would have been near impossible.

Mommy—Where would I be without you? You are truly the silent partner in any venture I have ever undertaken. You always know how to make things come together. You are the high priestess of tying up loose ends and smoothing out bumps. I would be completely lost without your input, guidance, wisdom and love. You are the Bon Jovi of mommies. I heart you to pieces.

Mark—You are the light at the end of all my tunnels. In this journey, it has always been your love, support and commitment that have made the difference. You are true blue, loyal, loving and consistent. Not even once, have you not been there when I needed you. I am humbled and grateful to have you by my side.

Carrie Frances—When I hear you say "auntie" all turns well in my world. I hope that one day you will look back at this space in your life and realize how much you inspired me. You are my niece, muse and mini publicist. Your perspective and brilliant mind keeps me focused. You motivate me to give the world my very best at all times. I am drunk in love with you my little sugar-bean.

Dr. Melinda Miller Thrasher—You are a genius. The first time I met you, you were sparkling. Your inner self was beaming with authenticity. Your practice is a ministry and a movement. Thank you for your thoughtful, honest, moving and spiritual foreword. I can't wait to see all the things God has in store for your big life. I love you and am forever indebted.

Ebony Steele—Thank you for allowing me to salute and uphold you on the back cover. It is clear that your fight with breast cancer only brought out what was already deep within you – unwavering courage, brawn and a ferocious will to live abundantly. You are a warrior crafted of "Steele," indeed.

Terri Jackson aka **The Connector**—You have the magical talent of seeing people's worth, inspiring with a purpose and helping like minds connect and collaborate. You have been my sister-friend for nearly 20 years and a soldier on the frontline of so many causes. Thank you for giving so much . . . all day . . . everyday . . . to everybody. Nothing is ever too good for you.

Dionne Battle and Plateau Events—I still cannot figure out how you manage to be in ten different places, at ten different times, doing all ten things at neck-break speed—with excellence. You extended your planning and coordinating services to me without blinking an eye. You made sure every resource in your rolodex became mine. You are sweet, supportive and always there. Thank you, my friend. I promise not to text you anymore at 1:00 a.m.

Justina Houston—God gave you the perfect last name, because your heart is the size of Texas. The way you feed into the lives of others is remarkable. Your venerability and spirit of service are both extraordinary and enviable. Thank you for your support, ideas, free counseling sessions and 25-years of friendship. You are so much more than a friend. You are a sister.

Teresa Wietzikoski—There is a picture of you and a tag of your name on the page of every milestone in my life. I honestly do not know how to thank you anymore. You have given so much, so often, so unselfishly. I am speechless. I love knowing (without a single doubt) that nothing has the power to separate what we share.

Phyllis Bryant—You are an amazing friend and confidant. Without any words being said you get me, and I get you. Our sense of humor is identical. I love it when we call each other and just seeing the other's name pop up, makes us laugh for the first two minutes—for no reason. That's love. You rock Phil.

LaToya Crenshaw aka **Lil' Mama**—I call you mama because you are the boss of the family. Your sweet, quiet, humble spirit is always fresh air to my lungs. You tell me the truth about me . . . all the time. I am so grateful for your consistent support, love and presence in my life. You always give the important and true things that money cannot buy. You are a priceless gem.

Jameca Barrett aka **SIL**—Some people are built for service, and you certainly fit the bill. You are an amazing cancer survivor and invincible warrior. I have never seen you hang your head once. In fact, I do not think I have ever seen you in a state that was not happy and beaming with enthusiasm. You are humble, driven, spirit-led, focused and intentional. Enormous things await you.

Genny Williams—You are my personal prayer warrior and supporter. You are 100% truth. No pretense. No ulterior motives. You only know how to be authentic and sincere. Thank you for always coming in HIS spirit to deliver an encouraging word or prayer that is unencumbered by the flesh.

Pamela Johnson—Eight hours? Really? Our scroll of inside jokes, joys and exchanges are enough to laugh a lifetime. You always say I make you look normal, but the truth is you really make me look normal. Thanks for always guiding me down the path of sweet sensibility.

Ros Williams—You are an anchor. You take on every obstacle in life as an opportunity to grow. Even when you are down—you are up. You are truly what Maya was talking about when she spoke of the phenomenal woman.

Reginald Christian aka **Twin**—Whether it has been four weeks, four months or four years since we last spoke, no connection is ever lost. You are dead center of what true friendship looks like. You are the mayor of steadfast supporters. I gotcha back! Club Candlewood, Regency Park, Sahara Desert or bust!

My Family Circus—My big clan of aunts, uncles, cousins and loved ones overwhelm me with the love and support necessary to soar, and at the same time stay grounded to the earth. I take none of your sacrifices for granted. I appreciate your support so much more than I can articulate.

IshNation—Social media followers, (IshNation Blog, Facebook, Twitter, Pinterest) you are the pulse and heartbeat of the 'Ish series. I write, you dish and keep the books relevant. There is no possible way I could achieve any level of success without your following and backing. You made me a #1 bestselling author, and I will always hold a special place for you in my heart.

Book Collaborators

Tony Smart—Thank you for a great back cover photo. You always bring the glam factor.

Ted Ruybal—You designed an incredible book cover that was true to my vision and cause. I pray there will be many more.

Ishpiration Auction Donors

Thank you for your dedications. Your financial support will contribute to nonprofit efforts to increase awareness.

Dionne Battle, Pamela V. Johnson, Vickie Mitchell, Janice Smoots, Dr. Sylvia Wright, Dell Smart, Belinda and Reginald Burney, Jean Scott, Genny Williams, Denna Porter Crutchfield, Marie Barrett, Beatrice Walker, Faye Wimbish, Vivian Griffin, Reginald Christian, Dr. Cheryl Best, Curtis Parker, Traci Adams Parish, Terri Ewing, Vee Byrd, Biviana Franco, Billy and Chandra Briggs

Committed Sponsors
You are the true Ishpiration behind all I do

Peachtree Dermatology Associates,
Sylvia Wright, MD

Fevour Cosmetics and Dr. Yvonne McCastle

Soul Purpose and Nadine Thompson, Terri Jackson
and Cheryl Cormier

The Hank Stewart Foundation and Hank Stewart,
Gwen Mason

Freebooksy and Ricci Wolman

The Firm Radio and Billy Briggs

Stella & Dot and Tosha Vincent

Love, Hugs and K'ishes,
Regina

-Special Editon Note-

This special edition gave me more excitement and anxiety than any previous book in the series. I was in a constant state of anticipation wondering how you (the loyal readers) would respond to my quest to honor women and their battles against breast cancer.

As with the two previous editions, all of the Ish statements are written by me, but the dedications in this book are personally crafted by the thoughtful loved ones of breast cancer fallen warriors and survivors. I found many of the 'Ish's from VOL I & II to be worthy of sharing again, so I hope you will appreciate that I added them to this special edition. You will find that I have kept each previously used 'Ish number true to its original. This is the explanation for the wacky numbering in the first half of the book. It begins with 'Ish #27 (from VOL I) and skips around through VOL II, ending at Ish #299. The brand new 'Ish's begin at #306 and run to the end of the book.

I hope you will enjoy and be ishpired!

Foreword

Ishpiration #339

"Sometimes the best self-work is done in the darkest hours."

Born in Harlem, as one of seven brothers and sisters and raised by a single mother, I learned early and first hand of struggle. My humble childhood surroundings made living through hardships as normal as a walk in the park.

When I look back over my life, I credit my mother, grandmother and the Lord for my perseverance, but it was my older brother who provided the exposure and guidance that resulted in my decision to pursue medicine. I studied Biology and Nutritional Sciences at Cornell University and graduated with distinction in all subjects.

I specifically focused my studies on obstetrics and gynecology so that I might have an early influence on young women's health and a life-long impact on the children they bear. Further, realizing that healthy lifestyle practices are best started young, I conceived "Before, During & After, LLC" in 2006. As a doctor whose practice is geared toward caring for women, it is clear that women are the central decision makers of their households, especially where nutrition, health and exercise are concerned. "Before, During & After" is the vehicle that allows me to share my medical knowledge through a speaking platform. I offer myself as a speaker to anyone who will listen: conferences, churches, health fairs, community and civic organizations. My ultimate mission is to empower women by educating, informing and providing resources that will enable them to make sound medical choices. It is this type of support that enriches women's lives and enables them to have a positive and life-long impact on their health, families and communities.

As a woman, I have a great deal in common with the patients in my care. It makes me proud to share a personal and professional interest in their lives. In practicing medicine over the past 22 years, I have undoubtedly learned as much from my patients as they have from me. There have been so many bright "ah-ha" moments. As an obstetrician, I can attest to there not being a more joyful and blessed feeling than bringing life into the world. However, the moments when I have felt my true calling and purpose for being placed on this earth were the times that were not so bright and happy. There have been innumerable times when I had to deliver bad news, bleak prognoses or walk patients through scenarios with high likelihood of unfavorable outcomes. Although, happy experiences make up the vast majority of my patient interactions, I think any physician would agree they are not the only prominent moments that rest in the memory.

I have grown infinitely from experiences where I stood in the gap with my patients and their families—all leaning on the strength of a higher power. I remember so many vulnerable times when I would look to the heavens and ask why or why not. Such times forced me not only to rely on my medical education, professional experience and training - but more importantly—my faith. WWJD? What would I want for myself or my mother?

In 2011, breast cancer's death rate for women in the United States was estimated at almost 40,000. It affects one in every eight—that is about 12 percent of American women. Conversely, the data for breast cancer survivors in 2011 is estimated at about 2.5 million. Annual testing will drastically reduce breast cancer's death rate and increase its survivors.

Heightened awareness and quick action can greatly contribute to your lifespan. Stand firm in knowing that a better and healthier life for you is a better life for your children and family. Annual preventive care visits, like breast and pelvic exams are a necessity. Consistent pap smear testing has led to a dramatic decline in cervical cancer amongst women in the United States. In likeness, early detection of breast cancer is linked to the decline of its related death rate.

One of the simplest ways to support and make each other account-able is starting a partner or buddy system with someone. Call your partner on or around her birthday—every year—to assure she has had an annual pap and mammogram. Make your partner account-able, and tag along on her doctor's visit, if necessary. Support each other's survival through increased awareness, consistent screening, early detection and treatment advances.

I am the product and culmination of all the sweet, bitter, life and death experiences that my years of practice have placed before me. I have learned that the most important work one can do on oneself is building faith, self-confidence, love of self and a foundation of spiri-tuality. When you find your best self, it allows you to be of greater service to others, especially your children. Regrettably, it is not dur-ing times of comfort when these vital traits come to matter, but in the moments of stress, turmoil and struggle. My husband often reminds me that a diamond is formed by intense pressure. I have witnessed my patients suffer through bleak times, but I've also seen them rise as bright and brilliant as a diamond. When women find their best selves they begin to shine and rise again. Remember, you are your family's greatest asset.

We have all survived some unfortunate circumstance. Thus, we are all survivors. So, in memoriam and celebration of all women (God's most beautiful creation) my prescription is for you to always allow your truest inner self to be revealed.

God Bless and 'Ishful reading to you all,
Melinda Miller Thrasher, MD—*Atlanta's Top Doctor*

Dr. Melinda Miller Thrasher is an esteemed medical practitioner, specializing in obstetrical and gynecologic care in Atlanta, Georgia. Her many distinctions include: Atlanta Magazine's—"Top Doctor" (2009, 2010, 2011 and 2012), Patient's Choice Award (2008 and 2009), Essence Magazine's—"Gynecologists You Love" accolade and The International Association of Obstetricians and Gynecologists—"Top Obstetrician and Gynecologist" honor.

Find out more about Dr. Melinda Miller Thrasher and her practice by contacting her at **atlantastopdoc@yahoo.com.**

'ISH—(n.) ish

1. A random, eclectic statement intended to provoke emotion—whether laughter, frustration, happiness or angst

2. Statement creating a gust of thought

3. A wanton expression or point of view

'ISHues—(n.) ish-oos

1. Subjects of significant concern

2. Matters of arguable debate

3. Hot topics

ISHpiration—(n.) ish-per-ra-shen

1. An eclectic statement intended to inspire

2. Words that move and incite positive action

3. The act of encouraging and motivating

'Ishpiration #27

Support a worthy cause with your time
...and money.

In Memoriam and Celebration of Life for

All Breast Cancer Warriors

Your life will always stand as a testament of greatness. No disease has the power to derail God's course or purpose for you. Share the trials and triumphs of your story to increase awareness and save lives. You are more than a conqueror.

Turn your pain into passion,
The Griffin Scott Press Family

'Ishpiration #29

Save $10 a week for your child's future.
If you don't have a child,
save for another in need.

'Ishpiration #31

Utilize the laws of attraction
to battle depression. Command that things

are already
as you would have them.

'Ishpiration #33

Start a nonprofit.
It's the ultimate way of supporting
a cause dear to your heart.

'Ishpiration #34

Once a month,
spend a whole
Sunday in bed . . .
watching old movies.

'Ishpiration #39

Forgiveness is for you,
NOT
the offender.

Ishpiration #41

Never refer to yourself as a victim.

If you're still living,

you're a survivor.

In Celebration of

Sonia Ellis-Taylor

Sonia is a proud member of the Church of Christ, Delta Sigma Theta Sorority and a tireless advocate for breast cancer awareness and research. She has a deep and authentic passion for helping, empowering and uplifting women. Her pride and courage as a survivor allows her to share her story and plight as an inspiration to others.

Your friend,
Pamela V. Johnson

'Ishpiration #44

Create a legacy to leave for your children,

even if it's just a lemonade stand.

In Celebration of

Leslie Burney

Leslie is an awesome mom, grandmother and mother-in-law. She is an outgoing and hardworking entrepreneur, who loves cooking and spending time with her grandchildren. She continues to support efforts for finding the cure.

**Your loving family,
Reginald, Belinda, Riana & Rashana Burney**

'Ishpiration #48

In your lifetime,
walk a mile,
on a beautiful, sandy beach . . .

in another country.

'Ishpiration #49

Drink champagne
with your
turkey sandwich.

'Ishpiration #57

Do *today*,
all that you should have done

yesterday.
and may not have the chance to do

tomorrow.

In Celebration of

Jennifer Carson

Jennifer is a retired educator, who truly is young at heart. In spite of battling the disease, Jennifer went on to earn a real estate license and launch an interior design business. When she is not designing, she is traveling—not wasting a moment or missing out on LIFE!

Love always,
Terri Carson

'Ishpiration #59

Hold hands

with your sweetheart . . .

in bed . . .

under the covers.

Ishpiration #60

Use *kindness* to *make a difference*
in the life of every stranger you encounter.

In Celebration of

Breast Cancer Warriors

One day God knocked on my heart, and I clearly realized it is better to give than to receive. With every gift "Box of Love," we deliver a much needed smile. With every box, we celebrate the courage of those who keep their heads held high. With every box, we honor those who battle the enemy we know as cancer. With every box, we pray that one day there will be a cure.

Feel Beautiful Today,
Biviana Franco

'Ishpiration #61

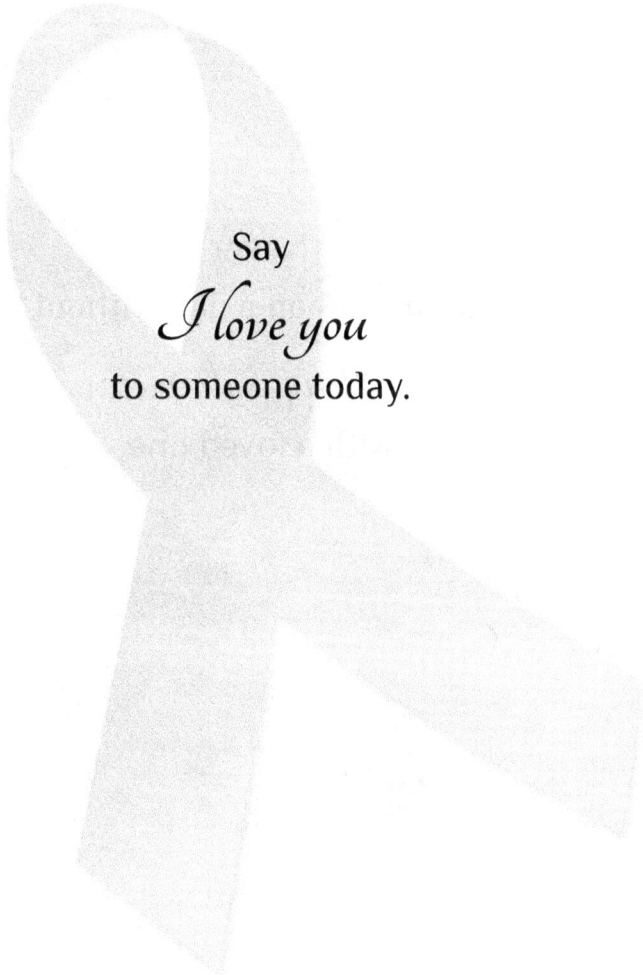

Say

I love you

to someone today.

'Ishpiration #63

Never
go more than a day without
settling a dispute
with a loved one.

'Ishpiration #68

Give in abundance,
even in your lack.

In Memoriam of
Mattie Sue Williams 1932–1964
Mattie was an Etta James fan who loved to dance. Her treasured gift of life was the first and last thing she gave. Her melody has stopped playing, but her dance of love continues.

Your daughter,
Rosalyn Williams

'*Ishpiration* #69

Relish a sun rising and setting

at least once a week.

'Ishpiration #70

In relationships, concentrate on
memories and quality,
not
titles or quantity.

'Ishpiration #71

Do all the things
people tell you are
impossible.

In Celebration of
Gina Seon May

Gina is a real life warrior and super-woman. She is the super mom of three college educated women, a super cook and a super friend to so many. In her worst moments she is still focused on giving to and enriching the lives of others. She is a courageous fighter, and still continues to beat the odds with style and grace.

Your friend,
Vee Byrd

'Ishpiration #73

Worship
a power
higher than you.

In Celebration of
Rose Smith

Rose has a name that is perfectly suited for her personality and manner. She is known for her fragrant hugs and sweet kisses. As a mother, she is always in full bloom and ready to spread an abundance of love, and as a grandmother she is soft, sensitive and delicate. She is a blessing to all.

Love always,
Jean Scott

'Ishpiration #85

Find the teacher who made a difference
in your life and
thank him or her.

'Ishpiration #97

Give 90 percent
to the world, but always
save 10 percent of you . . .
just for you.

'Ishpiration #98

Work hard and travel the four corners
of the world.

Rest when you die.

'Ishpiration #100

Don't wait for the perfect time to get married
and have children.
There isn't one.

'Ishpiration #102

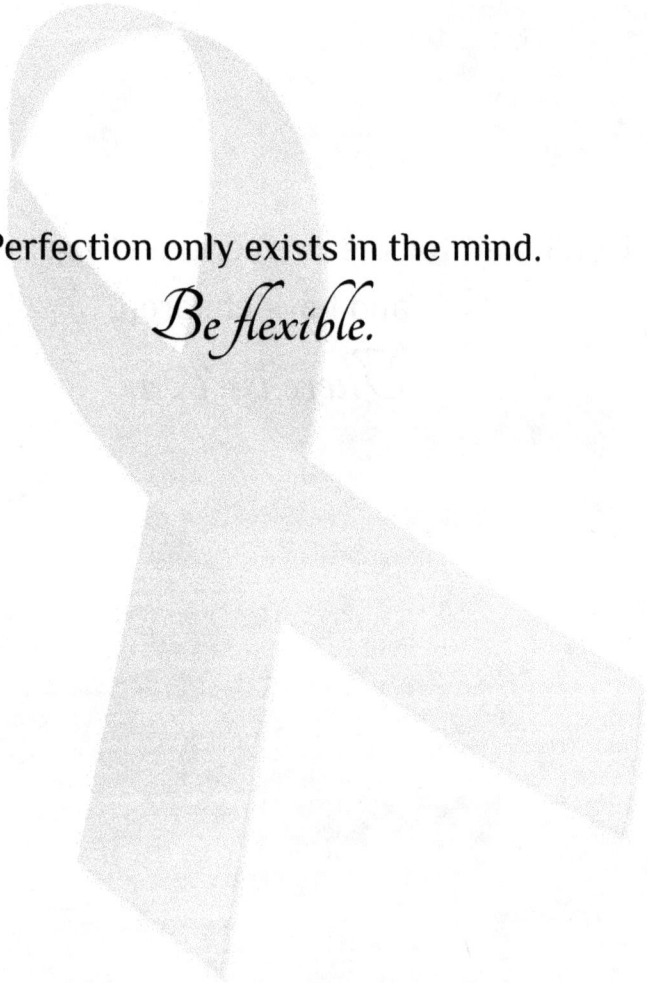

Perfection only exists in the mind.

Be flexible.

'Ishpiration #111

Give your
sweetheart
the last piece of
your favorite dish.

'Ishpiration #114

Coincidences and luck
don't exist, only
fate and blessings.

'Ishpiration #125

Smile and hug
more than you
frown and argue.

'Ishpiration #133

Drive your dream car.
You only live once.

'Ishpiration #134

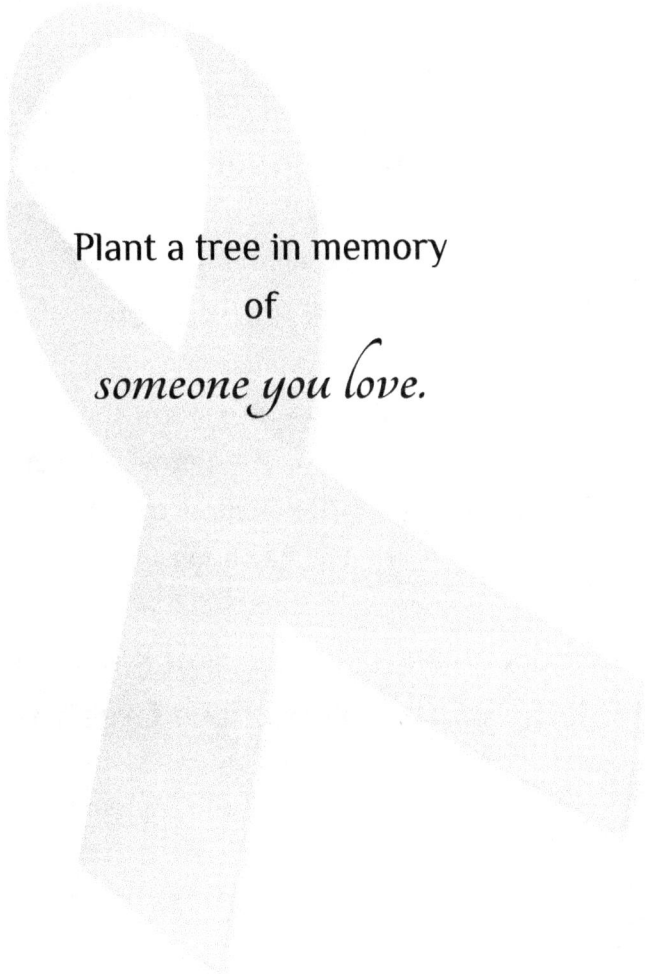

Plant a tree in memory

of

someone you love.

'Ishpiration #135

Remember the richness
in the sound of your parent's voice

In Celebration of
Gloria Jean Green

Gloria is a devoted mother who has given abundantly to her children, even in the midst of her own storm and illnesses. She has been cancer-free for over 10–years. Her will to fight and persevere has instilled the strength in her children to overcome any obstacles life may bring.

**God's blessings upon you & love always,
Jeffery Green & Michelle Green-Brown**

'Ishpiration #137

Buy timeless music,
and
play it loudly.

'Ishpiration #140

Chronicle precious memories
with pictures.
You can never have too many.

'Ishpiration #142

Keep a journal of your life,
so your children's children
will know you.

'Ishpiration #146

Cry often to cleanse.

Laugh even more to heal.

'Ishpiration #148

Living in truth
is the ultimate act of bravery.

'Ishpiration #157

Happiness is a gift
only you
can give yourself.

Ishpiration #158

Always give people credit for their
intentions,

not outcomes.

'Ishpiration #169

If one person has done it,
it is not impossible.
*If no one has done it,
make it possible.*

'Ishpiration #172

Luck
is where
purpose meets *destiny.*

'*Ishpiration* #173

The gift of giving
is rooted in abandoning all
expectations
to receive.

'Ishpiration #174

Live Now!
Every life has an **expiration** date.

In Celebration of
Geraldine Lester

Geraldine is a devoted mother, wife, grandmother and breast cancer survivor. She unselfishly and passionately enriches the lives of others through her life-long career as a nurse. She is a nurturing, tender soul—filled with grace and love.

You are a beautiful queen,
Anthony Lester

'Ishpiration #191

**RECIPE FOR A SUCCESSFUL
RELATIONSHIP:**
One pulls.
The other stretches.

Both Grow!

'Ishpiration #200

Stop wishing!
Start expecting!

'Ishpiration #206

A solid relationship
is like a good bowl of
sweet and sour soup.
The
bitter elements
make the
sweet even better.

'Ishpiration #208

Live a life that
makes the world
miss you when you are gone.

'Ishpiration #229

You can't sail the seven seas . . .
if you don't leave the safety
of the shores.

'Ishpiration #238

End all things good . . .
especially relationships.

Ishpiration #243

Leave the world your very best.
Die empty.

In Memoriam of
Bobby Jean Smith 1951–2011

Bobby Jean was loving, giving and supportive to all she encountered. She dedicated her life to serving others through the advancement of mankind. She worked passionately with the Correction Center for Women to provide hope to the incarcerated and homeless.

Gone but never forgotten,
Hank Stewart

'Ishpiration #252

Every life has significant
meaning.
FIND YOURS!

'Ishpiration #259

The world is bigger than your front door.
Explore other countries, cultures, races and religions.

'Ishpiration #261

Learn to speak the unwritten language
of the generations
before and after yours.

Ishpiration #262

Submission to **God**
is
PROTECTION from **God**.

In Celebration of
Felicia Payton

Felicia is an entrepreneur of great courage, faith and belief. Her positive mental attitude has her so deeply wrapped in her healing, she forgets to be afraid. She has triumphed over her vulnerability to reveal a woman who is poised, courageous and committed to her passion of educating others.

Your lifelong friend,
Joelle White

'Ishpiration #268

Your gut instinct is God's
whisper to you.
TRUST IT.

'Ishpiration #272

Change is temporary.
Transformation is permanent.
Ask a butterfly.

In Memoriam of

Yulieth Holguin 1932–2006

Yulieth is finally free. Like a beautiful butterfly, her essence will shine forever. Her love now has no limits, and her beauty is forever boundless. Her beautiful eyes will always see the light.

Your niece,
Biviana Franco

'Ishpiration #275

The past is gone forever.
The power lies in the present.

'Ishpiration #278

When you go through life in denial,
you can **NEVER** fully be the
person God intended.

Ishpiration #290

Wish. Believe. Pray. Wait.
Receive!

In Celebration of
Keva Hammond

Keva is an impenetrable rock. Her bound and determined spirit will surely kick cancer's butt. Though she is currently fighting the disease, her entrepreneurial spirit is still filled with passion and vigor. She personifies solid will and strong determination.

Your friend,
Reginald Christian

'Ishpiration #298

Rebuke the language of *lack:*
CAN'T . . .
WON'T . . .
IF . . .

'Ishpiration #299

Speak the language of *abundance:*

CAN...

WILL...

WHEN...

'Ishpiration #306

I can do all things
through coffee . . .
that strengthens me.

'Ishpiration #307

Leave a message.
I'm busy enjoying life!

In Celebration of

Lois Alexander

Lois is a proud educator and victorious breast cancer survivor. Her commitment to quality of life and community service keeps her entrenched in increasing breast cancer awareness. She is the epitome of style and grace. All who know her are inspired by her beauty and strength.

Sisterly,
Traci Adams-Parish

'Ishpiration #308

The most exciting part of
today is realizing the pain of *yesterday*
is behind you and the hopes of *tomorrow*
are before you.

'Ishpiration #309

People become skilled
at how to love and care for you by
watching how much or little you
love and care for yourself.

Ishpiration #310

Life places *roads* filled with
potholes in our *journey* so that
we'll *stumble* long enough to
realize our many *blessings*.

In Celebration of
Harriette "Johnnie" Davis

Johnnie has an incredible sense of humor and captivating personality that overflows with warmth. She teaches the importance of balance in all stages of life and instilled an appreciation for books, music, nature, family and so many other wonderful things in life. Our family has so many blessings from God through her.

**Love your great niece,
Sylvia Wright**

'Ishpiration #311

Make sure your daily multi-vitamin includes

500 IU's of *passion*,

1000 mgs of *faith* and

1 gram of *perseverance.*

'Ishpiration #312

The best antidote

for the blues is a

life-sized slice of cake,

topped with a pint of

Haagen Dazs ice cream

. . . **washed down with a**

carafe of wine.

'Ishpiration #313

When life deals you a
blow from the basement
of adversity,
respond
courageously from your
balcony of spirituality.

'Ishpiration #314

Dream *outrageously.*

Save *abundantly.*

Spend *wisely.*

Live *modestly.*

Pray *daily!*

In Memoriam of

Carole Ann Cooper 1949–2009

Carole wanted to celebrate her cancer's remission with an 8–day adventure to Hawaii. We swam with the dolphins, experienced a luau and captured life in its fullness. Our trip was a sampling of how she lived and loved.

**Your best friend,
Vee Byrd**

'Ishpiration #315

Even when things don't end like you
hoped,

*they always end as your
destiny intended.*

'Ishpiration #316

The four seasons of life are

birth,

denial,

acceptance

and death.

Each contributes to a 360° life

experience.

Ishpiration #317

Patience is what happens when you stop complaining.

In Celebration of

Ebony Steele

Ebony is woman of grace and strength who always manages to deal with whatever challenges life presents. Her "this too shall pass" attitude has served her well in the role of National Ambassador with the Susan G. Komen Circle of Promise. Her elegance and poise has and will continue to be an inspiration to others.

Love your cousin,
Curtis L. Parker, Jr.

'Ishpiration #318

Fear
never leads to greatness.
Faith does.

Ishpiration #*319*

A woman's life
is to God, as
clay is to a potter.
Both are molded and shaped
to create works of beauty.

In Memoriam of
Paula Anne Rolle 1952–1998
Paula was a blessing to everyone she met. Her faith in God was
ever apparent, especially during her battle with cancer. She had a
heart for serving, and was a great mother, wife, friend and woman
of God. Rest in peace my angel.

Your friend,
Denna Porter Crutchfield

'Ishpiration #320

Unconditional love
never
has an agenda.

Ishpiration #321

Positive expectations
are catalysts for
positive outcomes.

In Memoriam of

Madeline Enide Farmer, MD 1944–2009

Madeline was a loving and amazing mother, wife, friend and physician. Though petite in stature, she had a commanding presence that softly inspired excellence in all around her. She understood and taught how choices and expectations define our lives. She is loved, revered and appreciated as a true hero.

**Your daughter,
Sylvia W. Wright, MD**

Ishpiration #322

Expanding your horizons
is about overdosing on *foods,*
people, cultures and *ideals*
you secretly hate.

'Ishpiration #323

Authenticity . . .

is showing your true self, without fear
of repercussion or judgment.

'Ishpiration #324

There is no joy like that of a
solid,
happy
marriage.

Ishpiration #325

Dancing with your **feet** is about

expression.

Dancing with your **soul** is about

passion.

In Celebration of
Weader Simpson

Weader has battled breast cancer for five years, and is a true inspiration for women everywhere fighting the disease.
If ever you call her, it's like she's dancing at a dinner party filled with life and spirit. With Aunt Weader, it's never about her and always about others.

Love your niece,
Terri Jackson

'Ishpiration #326

Instead of allowing the universe
to drag you along,
have a say in how your life turns out.
The last word belongs to you.

'Ishpiration #327

Sometimes *life's sweetest* and most
treasured gifts
come in
tattered packages.

'Ishpiration #328

My NO means NO,
and my **YES** means I may change my mind
when I'm feeling better.

Ishpiration #329

Phenomenal—is part of the job

description of being a woman.

In Celebration of
Delois Malone

Delois is a one year cancer survivor, mother of three adult sons
and cardiac registered nurse. She has an appetite for travel and will
take any train, plane or automobile if it will end in adventure and
exploring new places.

Your friend,
Faye Wimbish

'Ishpiration #330

I'm not *bitter.*
I'm just cranky from all the work it took to
make me *better!*

'Ishpiration #331

I would prefer people talk about me
because I am
ridiculously bold
rather than
ridiculously dull.

'Ishpiration #332

Gratitude
for the
small things
in life prepares you for the
big things.

Ishpiration #333

Life is precious.
So, only use your fine china,

crystal and silver on days

ending in "Y."

In Celebration of

Lorraine Matthews

Lorraine is a courageous woman with an amazing inner and outer beauty. She is an extraordinary mother, wife, grandmother, sister, mother-in-law, aunt, friend and survivor. Her family feels happy and fortunate to spend the rest of their days experiencing new heights with her.

Thank God for you,
Terri, Steve, Halle and Stephen ll Ewing

'Ishpiration #334

Tell fear to
go
back
to
hell!

Ishpiration #335

Death does not have the power to kill,
strip, forsake or diminish the

love in your heart.

In Memoriam of

Stephanie Briscoe 1962–2004

Stephanie lost her fight against breast cancer at a tender age. She
loved the Lord immensely and directed the young adult choir in the
church where she grew up. She now sings in the heavenly choir,
most likely giving the altos the right note.

**Your God-sister,
Chandra Briggs**

'Ishpiration #336

The *world doesn't* define you.
It is you who *gives the world*
definition.

Ishpiration #337

The part of life before an illness is an
incubation.
The time during sickness is an
awakening,
and
the time of healing is a rebirth.

In Celebration of
Florence Obiako

Florence is two-year cancer survivor and mother of a beautiful
daughter, Christine. She is a generous and thoughtful soul, who
would travel the ends of the earth to help another in need. She has
worked as an educator for over 20 years.

Love,
Faye Wimbish

'Ishpiration #338

I said I'm fine!

The very next time you ask me if I need anything else, I'll be asking for a custom Bentley.

Ishpiration #339

Sometimes the best self-work is
done in the
darkest hours.

In Celebration of
Kathy Pavone Devine

Kathy is an optimistic and courageous breast cancer survivor.
She is a ray of sunshine, with a natural way of making people feel
good in her presence. Her strength should be applauded and stand
as an example that there is still lots of living to do after cancer.

Continued Healing,
Curtis Parker

'Ishpiration #340

Spend the weekend celebrating
life with loved ones
Write your chores an IOU.

'Ishpiration #341

In the midst of a
spiritual storm,
keep *prayer close*
and *faith even closer.*

In Celebration of
Aprille Maddox

Aprille is a living example that life is 10% of what happens to you and 90% of how you react to it. Her fortitude, thankfulness to God and positive thinking in the midst of the storm has served her well. Here's to cancer-free days for the rest of your life! I love you!

**Your line sister,
Dionne Battle**

'Ishpiration #342

You know when it's time to stop setting
goals and shooting for greatness
—you are dead.

Ishpiration #343

The most *powerful medicine* in the healing process is the *dose of hope* you give yourself each morning.

In Celebration of

Elmeta Brittion Matt

Elmeta is a loving, devoted mother and wife. She dedicated the majority of her life doing the greatest work on earth—raising her child and caring for her home. Her most cherished moments are spent preparing home-cooked meals, shopping, decorating and spending time with family.

**Your niece,
Vickie Mitchell**

ꞌIshpiration #344

On its own, bad news has
No Power.

It is only your response that gives the
news authority.

ʻIshpiration #345

Time has no refund policy.

Spend life doing the things

you love

with

the people you love.

In Memoriam of

Sallie Mae Johnson 1942–1995

Sallie Mae epitomized inner and outer beauty. Her kind heart and gentle spirit touched the lives of all she knew. She was masterful in instilling passion, resilience, loyalty and respect in others. Though, she was lost to breast cancer, her spirit is still alive and well in all of those who knew and loved her.

Your granddaughter,
Latoya Crenshaw

'Ishpiration #346

Speak **cautiously.**
Love **ferociously.**
Give **abundantly.**
Live **fearlessly.**

'Ishpiration #347

The
relief
to your suffering is hidden in the
silence and stillness
of your turmoil.

'Ishpiration #348

The space between life and death

is

your calling.

In Memoriam of
Bessie C. Phillips 1933–1985
Bessie was a faithful wife and supportive mother.
She proudly used her life to serve as a role model and dedicated
educator to the world. Her presence, humble spirit and mothering
gifts are deeply missed.

Love,
Belinda G. Burney & Don D. Phillips

'Ishpiration #349

Doesn't matter if you're smiling
on the outside, it is

the smile on the inside
that matters most.

Ishpiration #350

The only thing that makes you richer
than money
. . . is character.

'Ishpiration #351

Balance
is achieving harmony between
the yuck of yesterday,
the unpredictability of today
and
the promise of tomorrow.

'Ishpiration #352

Your worries should
never
be greater than your **prayers.**

In Memoriam of
Mary Bledsoe 1953–1998
Mary was an angel who believed in the power of paying it forward.
She took my boys into her home and loved and cared for them
as her own. She taught by being, doing and giving. I am forever
grateful for her gentle, caring and nurturing spirit.

I miss you,
Janice Smoots

'Ishpiration #353

Start your day with a healthy breakfast.
If not,
chocolate
will do just fine!

Ishpiration #354

Smile until your jaw *hurts.*

Laugh until your side *aches.*

Live until your soul *quakes.*

In Celebration of

Timolin Jefferson

Timolin understands the premise of being "battle-tested" and exercising every ounce of faith necessary to make it through a trial. Her perky and sociable spirit enables her to be a support system and advocate for others. She is a woman of deep faith and consistent action.

Your friend,
Dionne Battle

'Ishpiration #355

No matter how bad you think your life is,
there is always
someone . . .
somewhere . . .
in the world . . .
who would trade places with you to
better their own life.

'Ishpiration #356

Instead of focusing on the dark clouds
that come before the rain,

*anticipate the sunshine
that follows.*

'Ishpiration #357

I know you're tired, but you can't give
up!
Perseverance
looks so good on you.

'Ishpiration #358

Can somebody please give me a damn
hug???
Geeeez!

Ishpiration #359

People perish.

Memories live forever!

In Memoriam of
Christian Brown 1964–2011

Christian was an ambitious go-getter. He never met a stranger, and held a fervent love for his friends and family. He had a passion for entertaining and could turn the opening of an envelope into a full-fledged party at the drop of a hat. He fought hard and in the end—deserved his rest.

We miss you so much, your family & friends

'Ishpiration #360

When you find balance between your
work, passion and family, you'll be
amazed by all the
small, sweet, simple things
you never noticed.

'Ishpiration #361

When the landscape of your life
turns dismal, your spiritual fortitude
will make the difference in your
defeat or victory.

'Ishpiration #362

Humble beginnings

are fertile grounds for

abundant endings.

Ishpiration #363

I am *clothed* in power,

accessorized with grace,

& *scented* with the perfume of self-worth.

In Celebration of
Tricia Seraphine

Tricia is a dedicated wife, mother, avid reader, master gardener and awesome boss. She inspires others to be their best and do more with their lives. Even on her challenging days, she seems to find words that serve to encourage others.

Love,
Vivian Griffin & Rotonza Phillips

'Ishpiration #364

When you can't

Stand

the pain a second longer . . .

Kneel

and pray!

'Ishpiration #365

Trials and hardships happen in life to
build you
not
break you.

Ishpiration #366

Good sex
is like a shot of fine tequila.
It
calms the mind
and makes the body
feel good.

Ishpiration #367

The union shared
between a husband and wife
is the type of
rock that mountains rest upon.

In Celebration of
Esteban Jose Taboada

Esteban had the brave spirit of a fighter, even before being diagnosed with cancer. Since his affliction, he continues to show courage each time a new challenge arises. Eleven years of conquering new mountains as a husband is undoubted proof that the Lord Jesus Christ reigns. Thank You Jesus!

Your wife and friend,
Jeri Taboado

Ishpiration #368

Focusing on fears of the unknown

steals your

moment-to-moment

happiness.

Exist in the now.

'Ishpiration #369

Smile . . .
healing awaits you!

Ishpiration #370

You are
more profound and alluring than your
breast and
greater than the hair that crowns
your head.
You are woman.
Still.

In Celebration of
Julie Fuzell

Julie is a fun, wonderful wife and mother and brave breast cancer
survivor. If there is an event to be organized, she is the creative
planner who can pull it together. In spite of her adversities, she
continues to be a mentor to everyone she encounters.

Your friend,
Dr. Cheryl Best

'Ishpiration #371

Fight so hard
the
devil
has to call for back up!

'Ishpiration #372

Love doesn't mean you're blind to flaws.

It means they just don't matter.

'Ishpiration #*373*

Gratitude is always an acceptable
form of payment when your money
runs out.

'Ishpiration #374

Chance is what gamblers rest their
hopes upon.
Fate is what believers wait on.

In Celebration of
Sharon Bryant

Sharon is a high-spirited, humble, inspiring and courageous breast cancer survivor. In spite of the many obstacles her life has presented, she refuses to give up. She lives by the motto that she preaches "Lift up life, love living it and keep God first."

Your sister,
Dell Smart

Ishpiration #375

Who wants to live a

perfect life

when there is so much joy in living the

good life?

'Ishpiration #376

You can always tell when you

are growing . . .

it

hurts

like

hell!

Ishpiration #377

The measure of

good mothering

has little to do with all the

lessons taught,

but everything to do with

lessons learned.

In Celebration of

Angela Neloms

Angela is a brave and loving daughter, grandmother and wife of 26–years. She is a one year survivor of breast cancer. Her passion for life and work as an entrepreneur keeps her in the forefront of the breast cancer fight. She is focused and committed to educating women on the importance of early detection.

Love mother,
Judy Hutchins

Meet the 'Ish Master

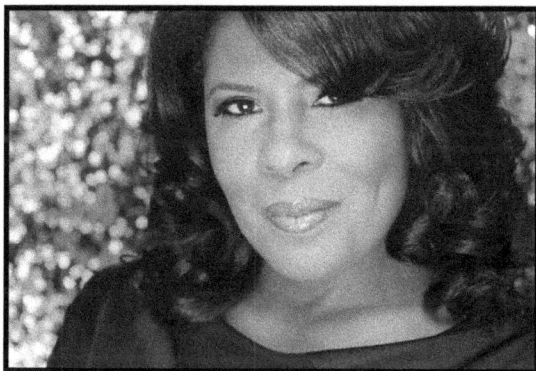

About the Author

Regina Griffin is a quick-thinking, life-loving, coffee addicted, shopping fanatic, lifestyle-indulging, social media guru. This Georgia peach and Atlanta native is the author of the bestselling, conversation igniting "Ish" series: "*Ish—Getting the 'Ish Out in the Open*" and "*Ishues—A Second Helping of Del'ishcious 'Ish.*"

She holds a Bachelor of Arts in Broadcast Journalism and has a tenured writing career that spans over 15 years—stretching from blogging to newspaper and speech writing. This author, publisher and entrepreneur enjoys connecting with readers through social media and live book signings.

Dish the Social Media 'Ish

Facebook at: www.facebook.com/ReginaGriffinAuthor
Twitter at: www.twitter.com/DishtheIsh
Pinterest at: www.pinterest.com/DishtheIsh
IshNation blog at: www.IshNation.com